Diagnosed, NOW WHAT?

A Guide to Navigating Your Cancer Journey and Embracing Life

C.R. Dismond

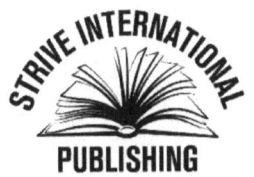

Copyright Page © 2025 C.R. Dismond

All rights reserved.

No part of this publication may be reproduced, distributed, or transmitted in any form or by any means, including photocopying, recording, or other electronic or mechanical methods, without the prior written permission of the publisher, except in the case of brief quotations embodied in critical reviews and certain other non-commercial uses permitted by copyright law.

ISBN: 979-8-218-83761-7

Edit and Layout by Shonell Bacon
Publishing Coach: Telishia Berry

Dedicated to my beautiful daughters: Sydney, Kaila, and Rachel.

Dedicated to my Special Sisters: Ericka, Stacie, Nicole, Natasha, Lisa, Kim, Nikki, Kahlia, Shonta, and Natasha.

Acknowledgments

I have so many people to thank for their contributions on this journey. This book would not have manifested had GOD not saved my life to share my story for HIS GLORY. The vessels of love, kindness, encouragement, support, consideration, advocacy, health care, education, and, most of all, prayers and just being present to talk or listen—I call these vessels daughters, sisters, bonus-mom, cousins, aunt, Spirit of Victory Church family, friends, prayer warriors, community members, podcast viewers, and capable caring doctors and healthcare team members.

Table of Contents

	Acknowledgments	i
	Introduction	1
1	Now What?	5
2	What Else Do I Need to Know?	22
3	Processing My Feelings	34
4	Faith and Fear, Can I Have Both Right Now?	47
5	Surviving and Thriving: Life After Cancer	58
	About the Author	66

INTRODUCTION

February 20, 2024, was the day I was told that the mass found at my recent colonoscopy was cancer. I was later told that the tumor was adenocarcinoma, stage 3 colon cancer.

I went completely numb. I waited for the stream of tears to start, but it never happened. I wondered what was wrong with me. *Did I really hear what I thought I heard? How did I get cancer? Should I be really scared? Is it OK to be scared?*

Even though I have faith in GOD as a healer, I couldn't help but to wonder: *Is this curable? Will I lose my hair? How will I look? Who can I talk to about this? Will people look at me and know I have cancer?*

Question after question flooded my mind, but the most pressing question was **Now What?**

Sitting, hearing but not listening as the doctor continued speaking, I bowed my head and asked God, "Now what?" Again, I felt like crying, but not one tear dropped. As a woman of faith, I did the one thing I knew to do and that was to pray. With my faith fully engaged, I looked to heaven and declared, THIS *story,* MY STORY, *for your glory God*, and I anchored myself with two Bible scriptures:

> *…for GOD has said, "I will never leave you; nor will I forsake you."*
> Hebrews 13:5

> *"For I know the thoughts that I think toward you, declares the Lord, thoughts of peace, and not evil, and to give you a future."*
> Jeremiah 29:11

I didn't know what was going to happen next, but I knew I needed to write it all down. So, I started a new journal to chronicle every conversation with my healthcare team, every question that arose afterward along with the answers, and how I was feeling mentally, physically, and spiritually every step of the way.

I'm a book nerd at heart, and I've read about all kinds of things, but cancer has never been one of them. I really knew nothing about cancer other than the negatives that I had heard. A need to know more about my recent diagnosis as well as a search for an organic way to help myself on the road to healing fueled my search. What I found regarding the different types of cancer, their occurrences amongst people of varying ethnicities and communities, treatment availability and accessibility, outcomes, insurance, and the costs associated with care—Boy oh boy! I was both enlightened and stunned. Again, fuel was added to not only my need to know more, but my need to help. I wanted to help others on a cancer journey answer some of the same questions I had, to encourage, enlighten, educate, and empower, and it starts *right here* in this little book.

Diagnosed, Now What?

Within these pages, you'll find questions to ask your medical team, words of encouragement, space to scream through your pen and paper and pour out your emotions while getting an infusion, reflect, make plans for the future, or to take notes while speaking with your physician. I hope as you travel the road to recovery that you are encouraged to keep going, and even when the way seems hard, KNOW that YOU ARE NOT ALONE. I'm here, like so many others, praying for you, supporting you, and cheering you on.

I wish you peace, clarity, and full restoration.

I AM A WARRIOR, ARMED WITH STRENGTH AND LOVE, FACING EACH DAY WITH HOPE, BRAVING EACH STEP WITH COURAGE, FACING EACH MOMENT WITH DETERMINATION.

I am relentless!

Chapter 1

Now What?

"Yet in all these things, we are MORE than conquerors through Christ that loved us."
Romans 8:37

First, **take a deep breath**!

Second, **ask questions**—lots of them!

Receiving a cancer diagnosis can knock the wind right out of you, leaving you with a heap of jumbled thoughts. Taking a deep breath can help you to pause and regain focus. Don't take breathing for granted. Those deep breaths may be all you can do to get through the next moment, treatment, or the overwhelming thoughts that continue to flood your mind. Again, I encourage you to breathe. Trust me, it helps.

CANCER DOES NOT HAVE TO BE A DEATH SENTENCE.

On the contrary, it can be an opportunity to regain focus of what's important and begin living life differently. How different may depend on the questions asked and the information obtained on this new journey. This is not a time when patients should worry about offending their doctor by asking questions. No question is off limits when discussing a cancer diagnosis and treatment options. You may gush emotions every time you think about your recent diagnosis. Don't apologize for being human. This is a normal reaction to receiving potentially life changing information. Fear of the unknown is normal, but I'm here to encourage you to anchor yourself in your faith (your belief in a being higher and more powerful than yourself) and tie a knot right there. Now's not the time to give up, but rather to fight like you've never fought before.

Get information, get understanding, and make the best decisions you can with the information you obtain. This is your diagnosis, your treatment, your journey, your life.

I've included information to help improve communication with your doctor as well as a list of questions to help guide you in conversations about your diagnosis and treatment plan. There is space after each question for you to write your answers for easy reference at a later date and perhaps use to encourage someone else. Because these may or may not be all of your questions, take some time to consider what else you'd like to know and jot it down on the blank pages following the questions.

Before answering the questions:

- Decide who you're most comfortable sharing this information with and take them to the appointments to help ask questions or write down information.
- Write down your most important questions before your appointment.

Diagnosed, Now What?

- Bring a notebook or recorder or use a recording app on your smartphone.
- Tell your doctor if you don't understand something. Medical vocabulary and concepts can be challenging.

1. Diagnosis Date: _____

_____

2. Diagnosis and Stage of Cancer:

_____
_____
_____

3. Can you explain my diagnosis in detail?

_____
_____
_____
_____
_____
_____
_____

4. What's the exact size of the tumor and location?

_____
_____

5. How did I get cancer?

_____
_____

6. Was there something I was doing that could have caused this?

7. How long have I had this cancer, and could it have been discovered sooner?

Diagnosed, Now What?

8. Can surgery totally remove the cancer?

_____
_____
_____
_____
_____
_____

9. Will I need chemotherapy or radiation?

_____
_____
_____

10. Should my children be tested? What is the likelihood they could be diagnosed?

_____
_____
_____
_____
_____
_____
_____

11. What is my prognosis (likely course or outcome of the disease)?

_____
_____
_____

_____
_____

_____

12. Should I get a second opinion? Where would you suggest I go for the second opinion?

_____

_____

_____

_____

13. May I have a copy of the pathology report (provides definitive information about the disease) and will you explain it to me?

_____

_____

14. Is there a treatment for cure or to prolong my life?

_____

_____

15. What are the survival rates with my type of cancer at this stage?

_____

_____

_____

16. What are my treatment options? Which treatment do you recommend?

17. How often will I have treatments?

18. How long will treatment last?

19. What are possible side effects and risks associated with treatment? How do I manage them?

20. What can I do to lessen the occurrence or severity of side effects?

21. How soon do I need to make a decision about treatment?

22. How will I know if symptoms I experience are from cancer or a side effect of treatment?

23. Which doctor(s) should I contact about symptoms and side effects?

24. To avoid confusion, what terms should I use when looking up information about my form of cancer?

25. What resources do you suggest to help me learn more?

26. How long will I need to be off work?

27. Will I be able to return to work?

28. What if I refuse the prescribed suggested treatment and go a more holistic route for treatment? Will you still monitor my health status?

_____
_____
_____
_____
_____
_____
_____

Over the next few pages, you'll find space to write additional questions you'd like to ask at your next appointment, make notes of information told to you by your physician or healthcare team, or even write out and practice what you will say when sharing the diagnosis with loved ones, co-workers, etc. Remember, there's no perfect way to have a conversation about cancer. YOU get to decide when, if, and how much you share. What's most important is that you feel heard and supported.

_____
_____
_____
_____
_____
_____

C.R. Dismond

Diagnosed, Now What?

C.R. Dismond

Diagnosed, Now What?

C.R. Dismond

I EMBRACE EACH DAY OF MY CANCER JOURNEY WITH COURAGE, HOPE, AND DETERMINATION.

Every breath is a reminder of my strength, life, and victories achieved.

Chapter 2

What Else Do I Need to Know?

Many are the afflictions (hardships and perplexing circumstances) of the righteous, But the Lord delivers (rescues) him from them all.
Psalm 34:19

No matter what kind of cancer diagnosis you receive, asking the right questions and enough of them about the disease, treatment, and many other things you may be wondering about can give clarity and allow you to feel less overwhelmed on your journey to recovery. If you think you haven't asked enough questions or feel like there's just more you want to know as you prepare to make some big decisions, pause and review the questions contained in this booklet. This could be a starting point to identify more about your diagnosis or treatment plan that needs clarifying.

NO QUESTION IS OFF LIMITS.

Make sure you've gotten enough information to answer the questions asked and that you understand those

Diagnosed, Now What?

responses. Be sure to ask your physician to explain medical terms, to repeat the information, or to even explain things differently to ensure your understanding.

1. Are there more tests needed to make sure the cancer hasn't spread?

___

___

___

2. Is this cancer hereditary?

___

___

___

3. Will this cancer or treatment affect my daily life? (eating, mobility, bathing, etc.)

___

___

___

4. Will my lifestyle change? (traveling, exercising, etc.)

___

___

5. Will I be able to have sex while receiving treatments?

___

___

___

6. Will I be able to have children after this?

_____
_____
_____

7. Are there changes that I need to make to my home environment while healing and going through treatments?

_____
_____
_____
_____
_____

8. What are the goals of my treatment? (to cure, shrink the tumor, etc.)

_____
_____

9. Are there any clinical trials that you haven't told me about?

_____
_____
_____
_____

10. Will I have limitations or restrictions as a result of the cancer or treatment?

_____
_____
_____

11. Will I be handicapped in any way as a result of this cancer?

_____
_____
_____

12. What are the risks of developing new cancers?

_____
_____
_____

13. Will there be testing or monitoring to discover if the cancer returns or if a new cancer develops?

_____
_____
_____

14. How will we know if the treatment is working?

_____
_____
_____
_____

15. How long will it take for me to get better and feel more like myself?

16. What can I do to stay healthy as possible during and after treatment?

17. What follow-up care will I need after treatment is over?

18. What are the financial costs associated with cancer treatment?

19. Are there resources available to assist in covering the costs of cancer treatment?

20. Are there resources to assist in covering other daily living expenses (mortgage/rent, groceries, etc.) while I'm off work?

21. What are some additional things I need to know?

Below, you can write more questions and requests you may have, along with the responses. You're building a reference tool that you'll be able to use to encourage yourself, and educate, encourage, and enlighten others.

_____
_____
_____
_____
_____
_____
_____
_____
_____
_____
_____
_____
_____
_____
_____
_____
_____
_____
_____
_____

Diagnosed, Now What?

C.R. Dismond

Diagnosed, Now What?

C.R. Dismond

I AM A PILLAR OF STRENGTH, COURAGE, AND HOPE, FACING EACH DAY WITH DETERMINATION.

I trust in my ability to navigate this journey.

CHAPTER 3

PROCESSING MY FEELINGS

The Lord is my strength and my shield; my heart trusts in him, and he helps me.
Psalm 28:7

There is no right or wrong way to feel after receiving a cancer diagnosis. You may experience numerous emotions all at once or one at a time for a long time. Feeling numb for a while or even being in a state of shock, are not abnormal, but knowing that other emotions will eventually come is important. You might begin to feel strong emotions suddenly, which could include anger or fear or maybe even grief and great sorrow. Allow those feelings to come and know they are normal responses to your situation.

    Acknowledging and respecting your unique process is essential for healing and support. Feeling unsure of when and how to talk about your diagnosis with others is not uncommon. You're trying to understand and be OK while processing everything that's coming at you and the decisions that have to be made. You get to decide if, when, and how much you share about your diagnosis, treatment, and your feelings.

Set boundaries. Be clear about the type of support you want and from whom. You can also set boundaries for any support you don't want, such as no in-person visits or no phone calls at this time. REMEMBER, there is no need for you to apologize for the boundaries you've set or decisions you made while trying to sort through your feelings and the information about your diagnosis.

Being heard and supported during this time is important to the healing process. Identifying who you feel comfortable sharing information with and having in your space during this very private time plays an important role in the recovery journey. You don't need to apologize for making decisions that give you comfort. Those who support and love you will understand.

While you may feel like you're on an emotional rollercoaster at times or that you're being flooded by emotions constantly, KNOW that it is completely human and healthy to FEEL what you are feeling. To suppress what you are feeling at this time could possibly cause undue stress, impeding faster healing and recovery time. Your emotions are unique to you, as are the cancer diagnosis, treatment plan, and overall journey. Don't minimize the importance of any part of YOUR JOURNEY, especially how you're feeling about what you're experiencing. To help make sure you don't minimize, I've included a few questions you may be considering that could add to the tidal wave of emotions you are experiencing. I also included a plan to get answers and understanding about the emotional part of your journey.

- What am I feeling right now?
- Am I allowing myself time to process my emotions while I also process information?
- What was I feeling yesterday?
- What am I most afraid of since receiving this cancer diagnosis?
- Who can I share these thoughts and feelings?
- What do I wish I could ask or say about my diagnosis that wouldn't upset or offend others?
- How do I share my diagnosis with loved ones?
- How much information is too much or too little to share?

Here's an outline to get you started on answering these questions:

Make a plan. Make a list of those people you want to know and also what you want to say to them. Rehearse it and read from it directly if it makes you more comfortable when sharing.

Find a good time and location. Think of the least stressful, most convenient setting where everyone is ready to listen. Try to include everyone you want to be part of the discussion so you don't have to keep repeating yourself.

Be as clear and simple as possible. Avoid sharing unnecessary details.

Talk about the process. Include what you've been told to expect in day-to-day life in your cancer fight and on the journey to healing.

Be open to questions and feelings and give them time to process this new information as well.

Use your support resources. Ask your physician for help in deciding what to share and how. Your physician may also be able to provide pamphlets or printouts about your disease and treatment that you can share with loved ones.

Stop when enough is enough. You get to decide what information you share, if you share, and when. This is your diagnosis, your fight, your journey. It's very important that your support system understand and value your need for patience and support while processing incoming information about your disease and the emotions provoked.

12 STEPS

Grieving the loss of health and your old life can lead to feeling powerless and hopeless or focusing on the worst-case scenario. Here are twelve steps to help you in processing and identifying what you're feeling. Remember, there is no right or wrong way to feel about your diagnosis. Your journey is unique, just as you are.

You Are Not Alone.

Shock and Denial. The first stage of grief is characterized by disbelief and numbness. The shock acts as a buffer, protecting the individual from the initial impact of the loss. Denial serves as a defense mechanism, allowing one to pace the absorption of the painful reality.

Pain and Guilt. This stage is marked by feelings of guilt, remorse, and regret. The individual may experience feelings of guilt for things done or not done, words spoken or not spoken. It's a tumultuous time when the emotional pain feels all-consuming, but acknowledging this pain is a crucial step in the grieving process.

Anger and Bargaining. This stage is characterized by frustration and annoyance. The pain of the loss may manifest as anger, which can be directed toward oneself, others, or the situation. Simultaneously, individuals may engage in bargaining, making deals or promises, often with a higher power, in a futile attempt to reverse or alleviate the loss.

Depression, Reflection, and Loneliness. Once the anger subsides, a long period of reflection begins, often accompanied by feelings of isolation and deep sadness. It's a time to contemplate the magnitude of the loss and its impact on one's life.

The Upward Turn. The emotional upward turn is a beacon of hope, signaling the start of the healing process. The intense emotions start to subside, and the individual begins to adjust to the new reality.

Reconstruction and Working Through. Here, practical and realistic aspects of life come into focus, requiring one to regain control and restructure life.

Acceptance and Hope: Embracing the New Reality. Eventually, the storm of emotions begins to calm, leading to a stage of acceptance and hope. In this stage, individuals come to terms with the new reality, learning to live with the loss. Acceptance doesn't mean forgetting; it means learning to live with the loss, allowing for hope and future planning to seep back into one's life. This stage is crucial for moving forward and finding peace.

Reconnection and Empowerment: Forming New Bonds. After acceptance, individuals begin to form new connections, strengthen existing relationships, and experience a renewed sense of belonging and support. Empowerment in this stage signifies the regained strength and confidence in controlling one's life and taking responsibility for one's healing journey. Reconnecting is essential as it fosters a sense of community and shared human experience, which is vital for emotional well-being.

Meaning and Purpose: Finding Fulfillment in Life. The next stage integrates the loss experience into one's identity and worldview. It's a time to reflect on life's values and priorities, to find fulfillment and purpose despite the pain. This stage is crucial for personal growth and development, allowing the individual to transform the pain into a source of wisdom and insight.

Growth and Development: Emerging Stronger. The journey of grief leads to a stage of growth and development. It's a time to recognize the potential for learning and growth from the loss and to transform the pain into strength. Individuals begin to see their resilience and capacity to overcome, learning to use the experience as a catalyst for personal development and self-discovery. This stage is pivotal for rebuilding a sense of self and finding strength in vulnerability.

Resolution and Completion: Achieving Closure. In this stage, it's a time to find closure, to let go of the pain, and to fully embrace life again. Achieving resolution means reconciling with the loss and finding a sense of completeness. This stage signifies the end of the grief journey, allowing individuals to live fully and love wholly, carrying the memories without the debilitating pain.

Forgiveness or Reconciliation: Finding Peace Within. In this final stage, individuals come to terms with their loss fully, often leading to self-forgiveness or forgiveness of others. This stage involves releasing any lingering guilt, blame, or anger and embracing a sense of peace and compassion. Forgiveness provides the final release needed to fully move forward without the weight of unresolved emotions.

Use the space over the next few pages to answer the questions from the beginning of the chapter and begin developing a plan to share information with loved ones using the outline following the questions. After, rehearse what you will say. Let the questions and outline act as a guide that assists you in identifying and processing your feelings, setting boundaries, and considering with whom you will share, when you will share, and how much.

_____

_____

_____

_____

_____

_____

_____

_____

_____

_____

Diagnosed, Now What?

Diagnosed, Now What?

Diagnosed, Now What?

I AM MORE THAN MY DIAGNOSIS.

—

I AM A MAGNET FOR MIRACLES.

Today, I fight fiercely and fearlessly—VICTORY IS MINE!

CHAPTER 4

FAITH AND FEAR: CAN I HAVE BOTH RIGHT NOW?

"I can do all things (even the hard, difficult, uncomfortable things) through Christ that strengthens me."
Philippians 4:13

Can a believer have faith and still experience fear? YES! This is why there are so many scriptures that speak about our experiencing the emotion of fear. God knew this would be a reality we would face, and He wanted us to be equipped for such times. Bible scriptures encourage readers when fear shows up; they gird you in truth—not to not worry or be anxious, to know God loves them with an everlasting love, to know GOD is the author and finisher of our faith, and to know God will never leave you nor abandon you. Below are a few Bible scriptures to that I pray will encourage you, empower you, and lift your hung down head when fear shows up and you think your faith has gone out the door. Use these to meditate on. Read them in the morning when you wake, read them aloud, let the words imbue you with peace, comfort, and fearlessness.

> *"For we live by faith, not by sight."*
> 2 Corinthians 5:7

> *"Faith is confidence in what we hope for and assurance about what we do not see."*
> Hebrews 11:1

> *"Have I not commanded you? Be strong and courageous. Do not be frightened, and do not be dismayed, for the Lord your God is with you wherever you go."*
> Joshua 1:9

> *"Do not be anxious or worried about anything, but in everything [every circumstance and situation] by prayer and petition with thanksgiving, continue to make your [specific] requests known to God. 7 And the peace of God which surpasses all understanding, stands guard over your hearts and your minds in Christ Jesus."*
> Philippians 4:6-7

> *"Be strong and courageous. Do not be afraid or terrified because of them, for the Lord your God goes with you; he will never leave you nor forsake (abandon) you."*
> Deuteronomy 31:6

> *"I can do all things [which He has called me to do, even the hard challenging uncomfortable things] through Jesus Christ who strengthens me (empowers me to fulfill His purpose for my life)."*
> Philippians 4:13

It is not impossible to live in faith and experience fear at the same time. We can have faith in God, God's plan for us, and God's plan for the world but still struggle with our very human fears. Be encouraged in knowing that no matter the state of our faith in God, His love for us is unconditional and everlasting and His faithfulness toward us is unwavering.

> *Lord appeared to us in the past, saying: "I have loved you with an everlasting love; I have drawn you with unfailing kindness."*
> Jeremiah 31:3

> *"if we are faithless he remains faithful,…"*
> 2 Timothy 2:13

The very word cancer is frightening. Illnesses like cancer may cause patients or caregivers to have doubts about their beliefs or religious values and cause much spiritual distress. It's not uncommon to question one's spirituality after receiving a cancer diagnosis. Cancer not only attacks you physically; it also tears at you mentally, emotionally, and spiritually.

The Bible is clear that faith does not mature and strengthen us without trials. Adversity is God's most effective tool to develop a strong faith.

> *"Consider it pure joy, my brothers and sisters, whenever you face trials of many kinds, 3because you know that the testing of your faith produces perseverance. 4Let perseverance finish its work so that you may be mature and complete, not lacking anything."*
> James 1:2-4

Cancer patients who struggle spiritually may no longer find comfort in coping strategies that previously brought them inner peace, such as prayer or meditation. Despite this, it is still vital for you to look to your support circle for the encourager, the faith speaking person, or the good listener. These people will represent a safe space to pour out what you're feeling and then be refilled with positivity.

Anyone can get cancer. So make peace with yourself and be gentle with yourself during the path ahead. Forgive and make peace with others, spiritually if not in person. Let go of past hurts and offenses. Now's not the time to continue investing in emotional baggage and pain that may be draining you.

LET IT GO, FORGIVE, AND LIVE.

Let's be clear, God did not give you cancer. God thinks thoughts of peace toward you and not of evil. Many patients may ask, "Why, did you let me get cancer, God? Why me?" Asking why is a normal response, but focusing on "Why, God, Why?" may get you stuck, frustrated, or even angry and depressed. View your diagnosis and the path going forward through the lens of scripture. Use scriptures to view your emotions, too. Every tear, all of your worries, doubts, anxiety, your questions of why, how, and what's next can all be held up to the standard of and viewed through scriptures accordingly. Take it one day at a time. You may feel stronger in your faith some days and not others. It's OK. These are times when you can call on your prayer circle or support that will speak life and hope to you. This will help you experience peace while moving forward in your cancer journey.

> *"For I know the thoughts that I think toward you declares the Lord, thoughts of peace and not of evil, to give you a future and a hope."*
> Jeremiah 29:11

Finally, develop your own personal spiritual care plan. Add new and different ways to feed your spirit (i.e., podcasts, YouTube videos, join a Christian support group, etc.).

FEED YOUR FAITH AND NOT YOUR FEARS.

In the next few pages, write down the things (offenses) you're holding on to that provoke negative emotions. Are you holding something against someone that is no longer alive, or you just don't talk to or see anymore? Write the name of the person, and IF you can remember the offense, write that down, too. If you start writing and run out of room, get more paper and keep on writing. Once you've finished, read what you've written, forgive that person and forgive yourself for holding on to it. Now finally, get rid of it. You're ridding yourself of the excess negative baggage. Give yourself to positivity and move forward accordingly.

_____

_____

_____

_____

_____

_____

_____

_____

_____

_____

C.R. Dismond

Diagnosed, Now What?

C.R. Dismond

Diagnosed, Now What?

C.R. Dismond

I'M NOT JUST SURVIVING;
I'M THRIVING.

I am a testament to the power of hope, resilience, and strength of the human spirit.

CHAPTER 5

LIFE AFTER CANCER: SURVIVING AND THRIVING

"And we know that all things work together for good to those who love God, to those who are the called according to His *purpose."*
Romans 8:28

Processing steps for navigating life after cancer may be just as overwhelming as when you received your cancer diagnosis. What's next? What questions do I need to ask now? When asking questions about your follow-up care, it's important to be prepared and proactive. Prepare questions to take to the appointments with the oncologist and your primary physician to discuss the plan after treatment.

Asking about the plan for follow-up care after treatment is important for understanding how to manage your health in the future. Your doctor might outline a schedule for follow-up appointments, tests, and screenings to monitor your health and detect any potential issues early. They may also discuss lifestyle recommendations and ongoing support services to help you transition back into life after treatment. This information provides reassurance and helps you maintain your overall well-being.

As you continue on the road to complete recovery and restoration, it's important to give yourself time and grace. Allow yourself the time and space to digest the very recent cancer fight and journey you've endured as well as the information and plan you've been given. Trust your instincts about your health, healthcare, and your journey forward. You are smarter and more wise than when you started this journey.

BE PATIENT.

Your healing journey has not concluded with the end of chemotherapy and/or radiation. Your body, mind, and spirit, and even your loved ones and support circle ALL need time to recover and be restored.

BE PATIENT.

Your journey after cancer is only just beginning. *Of what?* you may be wondering. That's for you to determine. Whether in remission or if all of the cancer has been removed and you're going into surveillance, there is a new beginning that will take place.

As you enter this next phase of life, regaining your strength and focus, I encourage you to take a few moments to reflect and also to look forward. I've included a few questions to consider during your reflection.

- What emotions am I feeling now that the cancer treatments have ended?
- What does surviving and thriving mean to me?
- What will I do now?

- How has my perspective on life changed?
- What will I do differently?

Take some time to think about those questions, then over the next several blank pages, write whatever comes to mind in response. If you run out of space, get more paper and keep on writing.

_____
_____
_____
_____
_____
_____
_____
_____
_____
_____
_____
_____
_____
_____
_____
_____
_____

Diagnosed, Now What?

Diagnosed, Now What?

C.R. Dismond

CHERISH EACH MOMENT OF LIFE'S JOURNEY.

About the Author

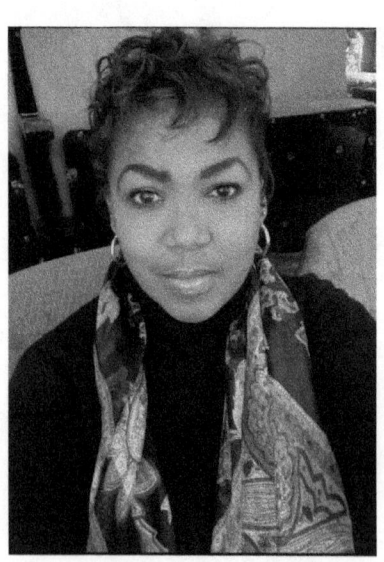

C.R. Dismond has racked up many accolades during her life. She's been a financial professional for almost 30 years, serving as vice president community manager for JP Morgan Chase-Flint, MI. She is also the founder of the Financial Empowerment Zone, chairperson for the Flint-Genesee County Black Business Expo, and a member of numerous committees and community focused boards.

What she didn't expect to also rack up was cancer.

February 20, 2024, forever changed the life C.R. worked so hard to cultivate. A diagnosis of stage 3 colon cancer, Adenocarcinoma, shook her world that day, but the question from her daughter, "Mom, what are you going to do?" ignited her quest for more information about colon cancer and her desire to connect and support others on a cancer journey.

Every story and encounter intensified the fire that has driven her mission to educate and bring clarity that helps dispel and dismantle the myths and fears that plague many fighting cancer. That fire fueled her to start the monthly online community conversation, Navigating Cancer in the Community, as a space for patients, survivors, caregivers, supporters, organizations, and healthcare advocates to have open, transparent, no holds barred, gloves off, wigs off conversations about cancer's impact on their world and life's journey.

Now, cancer free, C.R. is continuing to encourage, educate, and hold the hands of those who need to know they are not alone on this journey.

www.ingramcontent.com/pod-product-compliance
Lightning Source LLC
Chambersburg PA
CBHW071230160426
43196CB00012B/2460